The Ultimate Plant-Based Recipe Collection

Fun, Quick and Tasty Plant-Based Ideas for Family Meals

Levi Tonge

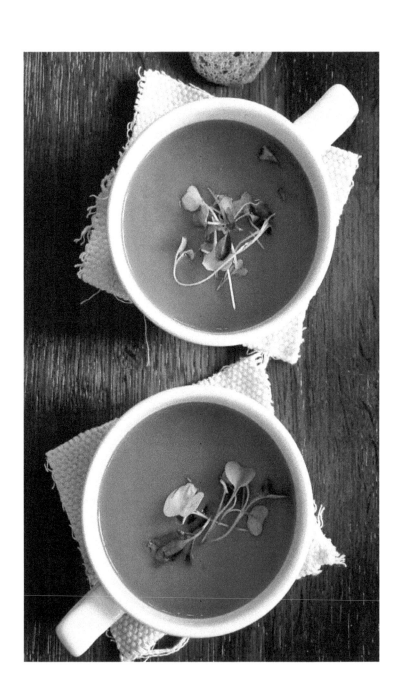

advice. The content within this book has been derived from various sources. Please consult a licensed professional before attempting any techniques outlined in this book.

By reading this document, the reader agrees that under no circumstances is the author responsible for any losses, direct or indirect, which are incurred as a result of the use of information contained within this document, including, but not limited to, — errors, omissions, or inaccuracies.

Table of Contents

Lemony Lentil and Rice Soup
Servings: 6

Cooking Time: 1 Hour 10 Minutes

Ingredients:

- 2 tablespoons extra-virgin olive oil
- 1 medium onion, chopped
- 1 medium carrot, cut into 1/4-inch dice
- 1 celery rib, cut into 1/4-inch dice
- 1¼cups brown lentils, picked over, rinsed, and drained
- ¾ cup long-grain brown rice
- 1 (14.5-ounce) can crushed tomatoes
- 2 cups tomato juice
- 2 bay leaves
- ½ teaspoon ground cumin
- 6 cups water
- 1 teaspoon salt
- ¼ teaspoon freshly ground black pepper
- 1 tablespoon fresh lemon juice
- 2 tablespoons minced fresh parsley

Directions:

1. Preparing the Ingredients

2.   In a large soup pot, heat the oil over medium heat. Add the onion, carrot, and celery. Cover and cook until tender for about 10 minutes.

3.   Add the lentils, rice, tomatoes, tomato juice, bay leaves, cumin, water, salt and pepper. Bring to boil, then reduce heat to medium low and simmer, uncovered, until lentils and rice are tender for about 1 hour.

4.   Finish and Serve

5.   Just before serving, remove and discard the bay leaves, and stir in the lemon juice and parsley. Taste, adjusting seasonings if necessary, then serve.

Curried Butternut and Red Lentil Soup with Chard

Servings: 4

Cooking Time: 55 Minutes

Ingredients:

- 1 tablespoon extra-virgin olive oil
- 1 medium onion, chopped
- 1 medium butternut squash, peeled and diced
- 1 garlic clove, minced
- 1 tablespoon minced fresh ginger
- 1 tablespoon hot or mild curry powder
- 1 (14.5-ounce) can crushed tomatoes
- 1 cup red lentils, picked over, rinsed, and drained
- 5 cups vegetable broth, homemade (see Light Vegetable Broth) or store-bought, or water
- Salt and freshly ground black pepper
- 3 cups chopped stemmed Swiss chard

Directions:

1. Preparing the Ingredients
2. In a large soup pot, heat the oil over medium heat. Add the onion, squash, and garlic. Cover and cook until softened for about 10 minutes.

3.   Stir in the ginger and curry powder, then add the tomatoes, lentils, broth, and salt and pepper. Bring to boil, then reduce heat to low and simmer, uncovered, until the lentils and vegetables are tender. Stir occasionally for about 45 minutes.

4.   Finish and serve

5.   About 1minutes before serving, stir in the chard. Taste and adjust seasonings if necessary, then serve.

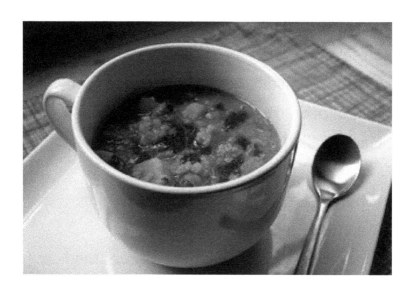

Matzo Ball Soup

Servings: 4

Cooking Time: 40 Minutes

Ingredients:

- 1 tablespoon extra-virgin olive oil
- 1 small onion, finely chopped
- 1 medium carrot, chopped
- 1 celery rib, chopped
- 3 green onions, chopped
- 6 cups vegetable broth, homemade or store-bought, or water
- 2 tablespoons minced fresh parsley
- 1 teaspoon fresh or dried dillweed
- ½ teaspoon salt, or more if needed
- ¼ teaspoon freshly ground black pepper
- Matzo Balls (recipe follows)

Directions:

1. Preparing the Ingredients
2. In a large soup pot, heat the oil over medium heat. Add the onion, carrot, and celery. Cover and cook until softened for about 5 minutes. Add the green onions and cook 3 minutes longer. Stir in the broth, parsley, dill, salt,

and pepper. You may need to add additional salt, depending on the saltiness of your broth. Bring to boil, then reduce heat to low and simmer, uncovered, until the vegetables are tender for about 30 minutes.

3.   Finish and serve

4.   When ready to serve, place three of the matzo balls into each soup bowl and ladle the soup on top. Serve immediately.

Miso Soup

Servings: 4

Cooking Time: 10 Minutes

Ingredients:

- 5 cups water
- 2 tablespoons soy sauce, or to taste
- 4 white mushrooms, lightly rinsed, patted dry, and cut into 1/4-inch slices
- ¼ cup chopped green onions
- 3 tablespoons mellow white miso paste
- 6 ounces extra-firm tofu, cut into small dice

Directions:

1. Preparing the Ingredients
2. In a large soup pot, bring the water and soy sauce to a boil. Add the mushrooms and green onions. Reduce the heat to low and simmer for 5 minutes to soften the vegetables.
3. Place ½ cup of the hot soup into a small bowl and add the miso paste, blending it well. Stir the blended miso into the soup and simmer for 2 minutes. Do not boil.
4. Finish and Serve

5.   Add the tofu and adjust the seasonings, adding a little more miso paste or soy sauce if needed, then serve

Tomato Gazpacho

Servings: 6

Cooking Time: 55 Minutes

Ingredients:

- 2 Tablespoons + 1 Teaspoon Red Wine Vinegar, Divided
- ½ Teaspoon Pepper
- 1 Teaspoon Sea Salt
- 1 Avocado,
- ¼ Cup Basil, Fresh & Chopped
- 3 Tablespoons + 2 Teaspoons Olive Oil, Divided
- 1 Clove Garlic, crushed
- 1 Red Bell Pepper, Sliced & Seeded
- 1 Cucumber, Chunked
- 2 ½ lbs. Large Tomatoes, Cored & Chopped

Directions:

1. Place half of your cucumber, bell pepper, and ¼ cup of each tomato in a bowl, covering. Set it in the fried.

2. Puree your remaining tomatoes, cucumber and bell pepper with garlic, three tablespoons oil, two tablespoons of vinegar, sea salt and black pepper into a

blender, blending until smooth. Transfer it to a bowl, and chill for two hours.

3.   Chop the avocado, adding it to your chopped vegetables, adding your remaining oil, vinegar, salt, pepper and basil.

4.   Ladle your tomato puree mixture into bowls, and serve with chopped vegetables as a salad.

5.   Interesting Facts:

6.   Avocados themselves are ranked within the top five of the healthiest foods on the planet, so you know that the oil that is produced from them is too. It is loaded with healthy fats and essential fatty acids. Like race bran oil it is perfect to cook with as well! Bonus: Helps in the prevention of diabetes and lowers cholesterol levels.

Brussels Sprouts & Tofu Soup

Servings: 4

Cooking Time: 40 Minutes

Ingredients:

- 7 oz firm tofu, cubed
- 2 tsp olive oil
- 1 cup sliced mushrooms
- 1 cup shredded Brussels sprouts
- 1 garlic clove, minced
- ½-inch piece fresh ginger, minced
- Salt to taste
- 2 tbsp apple cider vinegar
- 2 tbsp soy sauce
- 1 tsp pure date sugar
- ¼ tsp red pepper flakes
- 1 scallion, chopped

Directions:

1. Heat the oil in a skillet over medium heat. Place mushrooms, Brussels sprouts, garlic, ginger, and salt. Sauté for 7-8 minutes until the veggies are soft.

2. Pour in 4 cups of water, vinegar, soy sauce, sugar, pepper flakes, and tofu. Bring to a boil, then lower the

heat and simmer for 5-10 minutes. Top with scallions and serve.

Root Vegetable Stew

Servings: 6

Cooking Time: 8 Hours And 10 Minutes

Ingredients:

- 2 cups chopped kale
- 1 large white onion, peeled, chopped
- 1 pound parsnips, peeled, chopped
- 1 pound potatoes, peeled, chopped
- 2 celery ribs, chopped
- 1 pound butternut squash, peeled, deseeded, chopped
- 1 pound carrots, peeled, chopped
- 3 teaspoons minced garlic
- 1 pound sweet potatoes, peeled, chopped
- 1 bay leaf
- 1 teaspoon ground black pepper
- 1/2 teaspoon sea salt
- 1 tablespoon chopped sage
- 3 cups vegetable broth

Directions:

1.   Switch on the slow cooker, add all the ingredients in it, except for the kale, and stir until mixed.

2.   Shut the cooker with lid and cook for 8 hours at a low heat setting until cooked.

3.   When done, add kale into the stew, stir until mixed, and cook for 10 minutes until leaves have wilted.

4.   Serve straight away.

Nutrition Info: Calories: 120 Cal; Fat: 1 g: Carbs: 28 g; Protein: 4 g; Fiber: 6 g

Curry Lentil Soup

Servings: 6

Cooking Time: 40 Minutes

Ingredients:

- 1 cup brown lentils
- 1 medium white onion, peeled, chopped
- 28 ounces diced tomatoes
- 1 ½ teaspoon minced garlic
- 1 inch of ginger, grated
- 3 cups vegetable broth
- 1/2 teaspoon salt
- 2 tablespoons curry powder
- 1 teaspoon cumin
- 1/2 teaspoon cayenne
- 1 tablespoon olive oil
- 1 1/2 cups coconut milk, unsweetened
- ¼ cup chopped cilantro

Directions:

1. Take a soup pot, place it over medium-high heat, add oil and when hot, add onion, stir in garlic and ginger and cook for 5 minutes until golden brown.

2.   Then add all the ingredients except for milk and cilantro, stir until mixed and simmer for minutes until lentils have cooked.

3.   When done, stir in milk, cook for 5 minutes until thoroughly heated and then garnish the soup with cilantro.

4.   Serve straight away

Nutrition Info: Calories: 269 Cal; Fat: 15 g: Carbs: 26 g; Protein: 10 g; Fiber: 10 g

Classic Lentil Soup with Swiss Chard

Servings: 5

Cooking Time: 25 Minutes

Ingredients:

- 2 tablespoons olive oil
- 1 white onion, chopped
- 1 teaspoon garlic, minced
- 2 large carrots, chopped
- 1 parsnip, chopped
- 2 stalks celery, chopped
- 2 bay leaves
- 1/2 teaspoon dried thyme
- 1/4 teaspoon ground cumin
- 5 cups roasted vegetable broth
- 1 ¼ cups brown lentils, soaked overnight and rinsed
- 2 cups Swiss chard, torn into pieces

Directions:

1.   In a heavy-bottomed pot, heat the olive oil over a moderate heat. Now, sauté the vegetables along with the spices for about 3 minutes until they are just tender.

2.   Add in the vegetable broth and lentils, bringing it to a boil. Immediately turn the heat to a simmer and add in the bay leaves. Let it cook for about 15 minutes or until lentils are tender.

3.   Add in the Swiss chard, cover and let it simmer for 5 minutes more or until the chard wilts.

4.   Serve in individual bowls and enjoy!

Nutrition Info: Per Serving: Calories: 148; Fat: 7.2g; Carbs: 14.6g; Protein: 7.7g

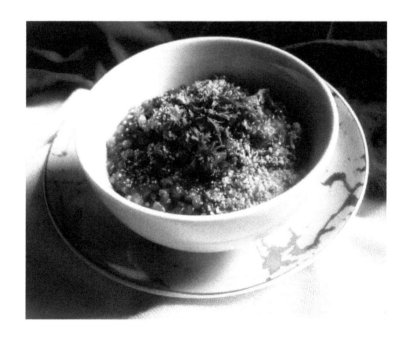

Fennel & Parsnip Bisque

Servings: 6

Cooking Time: 30 Minutes

Ingredients:

- 1 tbsp olive oil
- 2 green onions, chopped
- ½ fennel bulb, sliced
- 2 large carrots, shredded
- 2 parsnips, shredded
- 1 potato, chopped
- 2 garlic cloves, minced
- ½ tsp dried thyme
- ¼ tsp dried marjoram
- 6 cups vegetable broth
- 1 cup plain unsweetened soy milk
- 1 tbsp minced fresh parsley

Directions:

1. Heat the oil in a pot over medium heat. Place in green onions, fennel, carrots, parsnips, potato, and garlic. Sauté for 5 minutes until softened. Add in thyme, marjoram and broth. Bring to a boil, then lower the heat and simmer for 20 minutes. Transfer to a blender and

pulse the soup until smooth. Return to the pot and mix in soy milk. Top with parsley to serve.

Roasted Tomato Soup

Servings: 4

Cooking Time: 50 Minutes

Ingredients:

- 2 pounds ripe tomatoes, cored and halved
- 2 large garlic cloves, crushed
- 3 tablespoons extra-virgin olive oil
- 1 tablespoon balsamic vinegar
- Salt and freshly ground black pepper
- ½ cup chopped red onion
- 2 cups light vegetable broth or store-bought, or water
- ½ cup lightly packed fresh basil leaves

Directions:

1.   Preparing the Ingredients

2.   Preheat the oven to 450°F. In a large bowl, combine the tomatoes, garlic, tablespoons of oil, vinegar, and salt and pepper. Spread the tomato mixture into a 9 x 13-inch baking pan and roast until the tomatoes begin to darken for about 30 minutes. Remove from the oven and set aside.

3.   In a large soup pot, heat the remaining 1 tablespoon of oil over medium heat. Add the onion, cover, and cook until very soft for about 10 minutes, while stirring occasionally. Add the roasted tomatoes and broth, then bring to a boil. Reduce the heat to low and simmer, uncovered, for 10 minutes. Remove from the heat, add the basil, and season with salt and pepper. Purée the soup in the pot with an immersion blender or in a blender or food processor, in batches if necessary, and return to the pot. Reheat over medium heat if necessary. To serve this soup chilled, refrigerate it for at least 1 hour before serving.

Spinach & Kale Soup with Fried Collards

Servings: 4

Cooking Time: 16 Minutes

Ingredients:

- 4 tbsp plant butter
- 1 cup fresh spinach, chopped
- 1 cup fresh kale, chopped
- 1 large avocado
- 3 ½ cups coconut cream
- 4 cups vegetable broth
- 3 tbsp chopped fresh mint leaves
- Salt and black pepper to taste
- Juice from 1 lime
- 1 cup collard greens, chopped
- 2 garlic cloves, minced
- 1 pinch of green cardamom powder

Directions:

1. Melt 2 tbsp of plant butter in a saucepan over medium heat and sauté spinach and kale for 5 minutes. Turn the heat off. Add the avocado, coconut cream, vegetable broth, salt, and pepper. Puree the ingredients

with an immersion blender until smooth. Pour in the lime juice and set aside.

2.   Melt the remaining plant butter in a pan and add the collard greens, garlic, and cardamom; sauté until the garlic is fragrant and has achieved a golden brown color, about 4 minutes. Fetch the soup into serving bowls and garnish with fried collards and mint. Serve warm.

Broccoli Cheese Soup

Servings: 4

Cooking Time: 15 Minutes

Ingredients:

- 1 medium potato, peeled, diced
- 2 ribs celery, diced
- 1 medium white onion, peeled, diced
- 2 medium yellow summer squash, diced
- 1 medium carrot, peeled, diced
- 6 cups chopped broccoli florets
- 1 teaspoon minced garlic
- 1 bay leaf
- 1/3 teaspoon ground black pepper
- ¼ cup nutritional yeast
- 1 tablespoon lemon juice
- 2 tablespoons apple cider vinegar
- ½ cup cashews
- 3 cups of water

Directions:

1. Take a large pot, place it over medium-high heat, add all the vegetables in it, except for florets, add bay leaf, pour in water and bring the mixture to boil.

2.   Then switch heat to medium-low and simmer for 10 minutes until vegetables are tender.

3.   Meanwhile, place broccoli florets in another pot, place it over medium-low heat and cook for 4 minutes or more until broccoli has steamed.

4.   When done, remove broccoli from the pot, reserve 1 cup of its liquid, and set aside until required.

5.   When vegetables have cooked, remove the bay leaf, add remaining ingredients in it, reserving broccoli and its liquid, and then puree the soup by using an immersion blender until smooth.

6.   Then add steamed broccoli along with its liquid, stir well and serve straight away.

Nutrition Info: Calories: 223.5 Cal; Fat: 12 g: Carbs: 19 g; Protein: 10.6 g; Fiber: 1.7 g

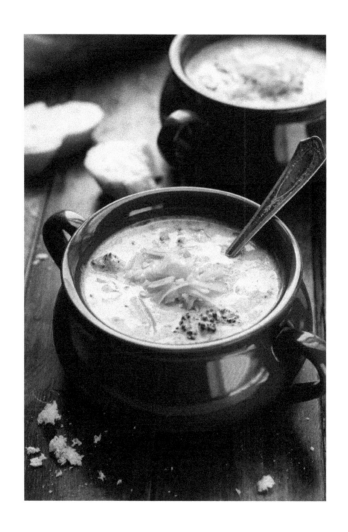

Creamed Potato Soup with Herbs

Servings: 4

Cooking Time: 40 Minutes

Ingredients:

- 2 tablespoons olive oil
- 1 onion, chopped
- 1 celery stalk, chopped
- 4 large potatoes, peeled and chopped
- 2 garlic cloves, minced
- 1 teaspoon fresh basil, chopped
- 1 teaspoon fresh parsley, chopped
- 1 teaspoon fresh rosemary, chopped
- 1 bay laurel
- 1 teaspoon ground allspice
- 4 cups vegetable stock
- Salt and fresh ground black pepper, to taste
- 2 tablespoons fresh chives chopped

Directions:

1.   In a heavy-bottomed pot, heat the olive oil over medium-high heat. Once hot, sauté the onion, celery and potatoes for about 5 minutes, stirring periodically.

2.   Add in the garlic, basil, parsley, rosemary, bay laurel and allspice and continue sautéing for 1 minute or until fragrant.

3.   Now, add in the vegetable stock, salt and black pepper and bring to a rapid boil. Immediately reduce the heat to a simmer and let it cook for about minutes.

4.   Puree the soup using an immersion blender until creamy and uniform.

5.   Reheat your soup and serve with fresh chives. Bon appétit!

Nutrition Info: Per Serving: Calories: 400; Fat: 9g; Carbs: 68.7g; Protein: 13.4g

Cabbage & Beet Stew

Servings: 4

Cooking Time: 10 Minutes

Ingredients:

- 2 Tablespoons Olive Oil
- 3 Cups Vegetable Broth
- 2 Tablespoons Lemon Juice, Fresh
- ½ Teaspoon Garlic Powder
- ½ Cup Carrots, Shredded
- 2 Cups Cabbage, Shredded
- 1 Cup Beets, Shredded
- Dill for Garnish
- ½ Teaspoon Onion Powder
- Sea Salt & Black Pepper to Taste

Directions:

1. Heat oil in a pot, and then sauté your vegetables.

2. Pour your broth in, mixing in your seasoning. Simmer until it's cooked through, and then top with dill.

3. Interesting Facts: This oil is the main source of dietary fat in a variety of diets. It contains many vitamins and minerals that play a part in reducing the risk of stroke and lowers cholesterol and high blood pressure

and can also aid in weight loss. It is best consumed cold, as when it is heated it can lose some of its nutritive properties (although it is still great to cook with – extra virgin is best), many recommend taking a shot of cold oil olive daily! Bonus: if you don't like the taste or texture add a shot to your smoothie.

Asian-style Bean Soup

Servings: 4

Cooking Time: 55 Minutes

Ingredients:

- 1 cup canned cannellini beans
- 2 tsp curry powder
- 2 tsp olive oil
- 1 red onion, diced
- 1 tbsp minced fresh ginger
- 2 cubed sweet potatoes
- 1 cup sliced zucchini
- Salt and black pepper to taste
- 4 cups vegetable stock
- 1 bunch spinach, chopped
- Toasted sesame seeds

Directions:

1. Mix the beans with tsp of curry powder, until well combined. Warm the oil in a pot over medium heat. Place the onion and ginger and cook for 5 minutes until soft. Add in sweet potatoes and cook for 10 minutes. Put in zucchini and cook for 5 minutes. Season with the remaining curry, pepper and salt.

2.   Pour in stock and bring to a boil. Lower the heat and simmer for minutes. Stir in beans and spinach. Cook until the spinach wilts and remove from the heat. Garnish with sesame seeds to serve.

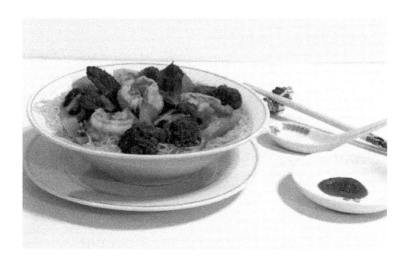

Farro And White Bean Soup with Italian Parsley

Servings: 6

Cooking Time: 1 Hour 20 Minutes

Ingredients:

- 3 tablespoons extra-virgin olive oil
- 2 celery ribs, chopped
- 2 medium carrots, chopped
- 3 medium shallots, chopped
- 3 garlic cloves, minced
- 1 cup farro
- 6 cups vegetable broth, homemade or store-bought, or water
- 1 (14.5-ounce) can diced tomatoes, undrained
- 2 bay leaves
- 1 teaspoon salt
- ½ teaspoon freshly ground black pepper
- 3 cups cooked or 2 (15.5-ounce) cans cannellini or other white beans, drained and rinsed
- ¼ cup chopped flat-leaf parsley

Directions:

1. Preparing the Ingredients

2.　　In large soup pot, heat tablespoons of the oil over medium heat. Add the celery, carrots, shallots, and garlic. Cover and cook, stirring occasionally for 5 minutes.

3.　　Add the farro to the pot along with the broth, tomatoes, bay leaves, salt, and pepper. Bring to boil, then reduce heat to low and cook, uncovered, until the vegetables and farro are tender for about 1 hour.

4.　　Finish and Serve

5.　　Add the beans and parsley, then simmer for 20 minutes, adding more broth if the soup becomes too thick. Remove and discard bay leaves before serving.

6.　　Ladle into bowls. Drizzle with the remaining 1 tablespoon of oil, then serve

Black Bean Nacho Soup

Servings: 4

Cooking Time: 30 Minutes

Ingredients:

- 30 oz. Black Bean
- 1 tbsp. Olive Oil
- 2 cups Vegetable Stock
- ½ of 1 Onion, large & chopped
- 2 ½ cups Water
- 3 Garlic cloves, minced
- 14 oz. Mild Green Chillies, diced
- 1 tsp. Cumin
- 1 cup Salsa
- ½ tsp. Salt
- 16 oz. Tomato Paste
- ½ tsp. Black Pepper

Directions:

1.   For making this delicious fare, heat oil in a large pot over medium-high heat.

2.   Once the oil becomes hot, stir in onion and garlic to it.

3.   Sauté for 4 minutes or until the onion is softened.

4.   Next, spoon in chilli powder, salt, cumin, and pepper to the pot. Mix well.

5.   Then, stir in tomato paste, salsa, water, green chillies, and vegetable stock to onion mixture. Combine.

6.   Bing the mixture to a boil. Allow the veggies to simmer.

7.   When the mixture starts simmering, add the beans.

8.   Bring the veggie mixture to a simmer again and lower the heat to low.

9.   Finally, cook for 15 to 20 minutes and check for seasoning. Add more salt and pepper if needed.

10.   Garnish with the topping of your choice. Serve it hot.

Mushroom & Tofu Soup

Servings: 4

Cooking Time: 20 Minutes

Ingredients:

- 4 cups water
- 2 tbsp soy sauce
- 4 white mushrooms, sliced
- ¼ cup chopped green onions
- 3 tbsp tahini
- 6 oz extra-firm tofu, diced

Directions:

1.   Pour the water and soy sauce in a pot and bring to a boil. Add in mushrooms and green onions. Lower the heat and simmer for minutes. In a bowl, combine ½ cup of hot soup with tahini. Pour the mixture into the pot and simmer 2 minutes more, but not boil. Stir in tofu. Serve warm.

Beans-and-rice Soup with Collards

Servings: 4 To 6

Cooking Time: 50 Minutes

Ingredients:

- 6 cups coarsely chopped stemmed collard greens
- 2 tablespoons extra-virgin olive oil
- 1 medium onion, chopped
- 2 garlic cloves, minced
- 3 cups cooked or 2 (15.5-ounce) cans black-eyed peas, drained and rinsed
- 5 cups vegetable broth, homemade or store-bought, or water
- Salt and freshly ground black pepper
- ½ cup long-grain brown rice
- Tabasco sauce, for serving

Directions:

1. Preparing the Ingredients
2. In a pot of boiling salted water, cook the collards until tender for about minutes. Drain and set aside.
3. In a large soup pot, heat the oil over medium heat. Add the onion and garlic, cover, and cook until softened

for about 5 minutes. Stir in the black-eyed peas, broth, cooked collards, and salt and pepper.

4.   Finish and serve

5.   Bring to a boil, then reduce heat to low, add the rice and simmer, uncovered, until the rice is cooked for about 30 minutes. Serve with Tabasco sauce.

Spinach, Tomato, And Orzo Soup

Servings: 6

Cooking Time: 20 Minutes

Ingredients:

- 1 tablespoon extra-virgin olive oil
- 1 onion, chopped
- 4 garlic cloves, minced
- 1 (14.5-ounce) can diced Italian tomatoes (preferably with oregano and basil)
- 4 cups low-sodium vegetable broth
- 4 cups water
- 1 teaspoon sea salt
- 1 teaspoon black pepper
- 1 pound uncooked orzo pasta
- 1 (5-ounce) package baby spinach

Directions:

1. Preparing the Ingredients

2. Heat the oil in a large stockpot over medium heat. Add the onion and sauté for 3 minutes, or until soft. Add the garlic and sauté for 1 additional minute, or until fragrant. Add the tomatoes with their juice, broth, water,

salt, and pepper. Cover the pot and bring to a boil. Reduce the heat to a simmer.

3.	Add the orzo and cook, uncovered, for 9 minutes, or until the pasta is tender.

4.	Finish and serve

5.	Turn off the heat and stir in the spinach until wilted.

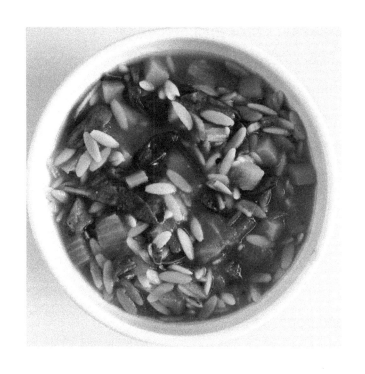

Balsamic Lentil Stew

Servings: 5

Cooking Time: 30 Minutes

Ingredients:

- 1 teaspoon extra-virgin olive oil
- 4 carrots, peeled and chopped
- 1 onion, chopped
- 3 garlic cloves, minced
- 2 tablespoons balsamic vinegar
- 4 cups Vegetable Broth or water
- 1 (28-ounce) can crushed tomatoes
- 1 tablespoon sugar
- 2 cups dried lentils or 2 (15-ounce) cans lentils, drained and rinsed
- 1 teaspoon salt
- Freshly ground black pepper

Directions:

1. Preparing the Ingredients

2. Heat the olive oil in a large soup pot over medium heat.

3. Add the carrots, onion, and garlic, then sauté for about 5 minutes until the vegetables are softened. Pour

in the vinegar, and let it sizzle to deglaze the bottom of the pot. Add the vegetable broth, tomatoes, sugar, and lentils.

4.   Bring to a boil, then reduce the heat to low. Simmer for about 25 minutes until the lentils are soft.

5.   Finish and Serve

6.   Add the salt and season with pepper. Leftovers will keep in an airtight container for up to 1 week in the refrigerator, or up to 1 month in the freezer.

Nutrition Info: Per Serving: (2 cups) Calories 353; Protein: 22g; Total fat: 2g; Saturated fat: 0g; Carbohydrates: 67g; Fiber: 27g

Leek And Potato Soup (pressure Cooker)

Servings: 4-6

Cooking Time: 15 Minutes

Ingredients:

- 3 leeks (white and light green parts only), chopped
- 1 white or yellow onion, chopped
- 3 or 4 garlic cloves, minced
- 1 tablespoon olive oil
- 6 medium russet potatoes, scrubbed or peeled and roughly chopped (6 to 7 cups)
- ½ (13.5-ounce) can coconut milk (about ¾ cup)
- 4 cups water or unsalted vegetable broth
- ½ teaspoon salt, plus more as needed
- 1 teaspoon garlic powder (optional)
- Freshly ground black pepper

Directions:

1. Preparing the Ingredients. On your electric pressure cooker, select Sauté. Add the leeks, onion, garlic, and olive oil. Cook for 4 to 5 minutes, until the leek and onion are softened. Add the potatoes, coconut milk, water, and salt. Cancel Sauté.

2.　　High pressure for 7 minutes. Close and lock the lid, and select High Pressure for 7 minutes.

3.　　Pressure Release. Let the pressure release naturally, about 20 minutes. Unlock and remove the lid. Let cool for a few minutes and then purée the soup— either transfer the soup (in batches, if necessary) to a countertop blender. Taste and season with the garlic powder (if using), salt, and pepper.

Nutrition Info: Per Serving: Calories: 274; Protein: 5g; Total fat: 10g; Carbohydrates: 75g; Fiber: 4g

Moroccan Bean Stew

Servings: 4

Cooking Time: 40 Minutes

Ingredients:

- 3 cups cooked red kidney beans
- 2 tbsp olive oil
- 1 yellow onion, chopped
- 2 carrots, sliced
- 3 garlic cloves, minced
- 1 tsp grated fresh ginger
- ½ tsp ground cumin
- 1 tsp ras el hanout
- 2 russet potatoes, chopped
- 1 (14.5-oz) can crushed tomatoes
- 1 (4-oz) can diced green chiles, drained
- 1 ½ cups vegetable broth
- Salt and black pepper to taste
- 3 cups eggplants, chopped
- ⅓ cup chopped roasted peanuts

Directions:

1.   Heat the oil in a pot over medium heat. Place the onion, garlic, ginger, and carrots and sauté for 5 minutes

until tender. Stir in cumin, ras el hanout, potatoes, beans, tomatoes, chiles, and broth. Season with salt and pepper. Bring to a boil, then lower the heat and simmer for 20 minutes. Add in eggplants and cook for minutes. Serve garnished with peanuts.

Cauliflower Asparagus Soup

Servings: 4

Cooking Time: 30 Minutes

Ingredients:

- 20 asparagus spears, chopped
- 4 cups vegetable stock
- ½ cauliflower head, chopped
- 2 garlic cloves, chopped
- 1 tbsp coconut oil
- Pepper
- Salt

Directions:

1. Heat coconut oil in a large saucepan over medium heat.
2. Add garlic and sauté until softened.
3. Add cauliflower, vegetable stock, pepper, and salt. Stir well and bring to boil.
4. Reduce heat to low and simmer for 20 minutes.
5. Add chopped asparagus and cook until softened.
6. Puree the soup using an immersion blender until smooth and creamy.
7. Stir well and serve warm.

Winter Root Vegetable Soup

Servings: 4

Cooking Time: 40 Minutes

Ingredients:

- 4 tablespoons avocado oil
- 1 large leek, sliced
- 2 carrots, diced
- 2 parsnips, diced
- 2 cups turnip, diced
- 2 celery stalks, diced
- 1 pound sweet potatoes, diced
- 1 teaspoon ginger-garlic paste
- 1 habanero pepper, seeded and chopped
- 1/2 teaspoon caraway seeds
- 1/2 teaspoon fennel seeds
- 2 bay leaves
- Sea salt and ground black pepper, to season
- 1 teaspoon cayenne pepper
- 4 cups vegetable broth
- 4 tablespoons tahini

Directions:

1.   In a stockpot, heat the oil over medium-high heat. Now, sauté the leeks, carrots, parsnip, turnip, celery and sweet potatoes for about 5 minutes, stirring periodically.

2.   Add in the ginger-garlic paste and habanero peppers and continue sautéing for 1 minute or until fragrant.

3.   Then, stir in the caraway seeds, fennel seeds, bay leaves, salt, black pepper, cayenne pepper and vegetable broth; bring to a boil. Immediately turn the heat to a simmer and let it cook for approximately 25 minutes.

4.   Puree the soup using an immersion blender until creamy and uniform.

5.   Return the pureed mixture to the pot. Fold in the tahini and continue to simmer until heated through or about minutes longer.

6.   Ladle into individual bowls and serve hot. Bon appétit!

Nutrition Info: Per Serving: Calories: 427; Fat: 24.2g; Carbs: 41.4g; Protein: 13.7g

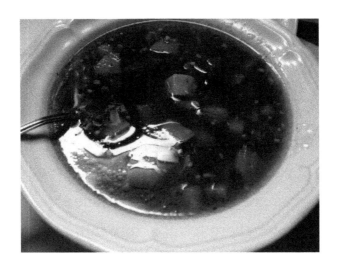

Winter Quinoa Salad with Pickles

Servings: 4

Cooking Time: 20 Minutes

Ingredients:

- 1 cup quinoa
- 4 garlic cloves, minced
- 2 pickled cucumber, chopped
- 10 ounces canned red peppers, chopped
- 1/2 cup green olives, pitted and sliced
- 2 cups green cabbages, shredded
- 2 cups Iceberg lettuce, torn into pieces
- 4 pickled chilies, chopped
- 4 tablespoons olive oil
- 1 tablespoon lemon juice
- 1 teaspoon lemon zest
- 1/2 teaspoon dried marjoram
- Sea salt and ground black pepper, to taste
- 1/4 cup fresh chives, coarsely chopped

Directions:

1.   Place two cups of water and the quinoa in a pot and bring it to a boil. Immediately turn the heat to a simmer.

2.   Let it simmer for about 13 minutes until the quinoa has absorbed all of the water; fluff the quinoa with a fork and let it cool completely. Then, transfer the quinoa to a salad bowl.

3.   Add the garlic, pickled cucumber, peppers, olives, cabbage, lettuce and pickled chilies to the salad bowl and toss to combine.

4.   In a small mixing bowl, make the dressing by whisking the remaining ingredients. Dress the salad, toss to combine well and serve immediately. Bon appétit!

Nutrition Info: Per Serving: Calories: 346; Fat: 16.7g; Carbs: 42.6g; Protein: 9.3g

Roasted Wild Mushroom Soup

Servings: 3

Cooking Time: 55 Minutes

Ingredients:

- 3 tablespoons sesame oil
- 1 pound mixed wild mushrooms, sliced
- 1 white onion, chopped
- 3 cloves garlic, minced and divided
- 2 sprigs thyme, chopped
- 2 sprigs rosemary, chopped
- 1/4 cup flaxseed meal
- 1/4 cup dry white wine
- 3 cups vegetable broth
- 1/2 teaspoon red chili flakes
- Garlic salt and freshly ground black pepper, to seasoned

Directions:

1. Start by preheating your oven to 395 degrees F.
2. Place the mushrooms in a single layer onto a parchment-lined baking pan. Drizzle the mushrooms with 1 tablespoon of the sesame oil.

3.   Roast the mushrooms in the preheated oven for about 25 minutes, or until tender.

4.   Heat the remaining 2 tablespoons of the sesame oil in a stockpot over medium heat. Then, sauté the onion for about 3 minutes or until tender and translucent.

5.   Then, add in the garlic, thyme and rosemary and continue to sauté for 1 minute or so until aromatic. Sprinkle flaxseed meal over everything.

6.   Add in the remaining ingredients and continue to simmer for 10 to 15 minutes longer or until everything is cooked through.

7.   Stir in the roasted mushrooms and continue simmering for a further 12 minutes. Ladle into soup bowls and serve hot. Enjoy!

Nutrition Info: Per Serving: Calories: 313; Fat: 23.5g; Carbs: 14.5g; Protein: 14.5g

Vegetarian Gumbo

Servings: 4

Cooking Time: 45 Minutes

Ingredients:

- 1 1/2 cups diced zucchini
- 16-ounces cooked red beans
- 4 cups sliced okra
- 1 1/2 cups diced green pepper
- 1 1/2 cups chopped white onion
- 1 1/2 cups diced red bell pepper
- 8 cremini mushrooms, quartered
- 1 cup sliced celery
- 3 teaspoons minced garlic
- 1 medium tomato, chopped
- 1 teaspoon red pepper flakes
- 1 teaspoon dried thyme
- 3 tablespoons all-purpose flour
- 1 tablespoon smoked paprika
- 1 teaspoon dried oregano
- 1/4 teaspoon nutmeg
- 1 teaspoon soy sauce
- 1 1/2 teaspoons liquid smoke
- 2 tablespoons mustard

- 1 tablespoon apple cider vinegar
- 1 tablespoon Worcestershire sauce, vegetarian
- 1/2 teaspoon hot sauce
- 3 tablespoons olive oil
- 4 cups vegetable stock
- 1/2 cups sliced green onion
- 4 cups cooked jasmine rice

Directions:

1.   Take a Dutch oven, place it over medium heat, add oil and flour and cook for 5 minutes until fragrant.

2.   Switch heat to the medium low level, and continue cooking for minutes until roux becomes dark brown, whisking constantly.

3.   Meanwhile, place the tomato in a food processor, add garlic and onion along with remaining ingredients, except for stock, zucchini, celery, mushroom, green and red bell pepper, and pulse for 2 minutes until smooth.

4.   Pour the mixture into the pan, return pan over medium-high heat, stir until mixed, and cook for 5 minutes until all the liquid has evaporated.

5.   Stir in stock, bring it to simmer, then add remaining vegetables and simmer for 20 minutes until tender.

6.   Garnish gumbo with green onions and serve with rice.

Nutrition Info: Calories: 160 Cal; Fat: 7.3 g: Carbs: 20 g; Protein: 7 g; Fiber: 5.7 g

Creamy Potato-cauliflower Soup

Servings: 6

Cooking Time: 25 Minutes

Ingredients:

- 1 teaspoon extra-virgin olive oil
- 1 onion, chopped
- 3 cups chopped cauliflower
- 2 potatoes, scrubbed or peeled and chopped
- 6 cups water or Vegetable Broth
- 2 tablespoons dried herbs
- Salt
- Freshly ground black pepper
- 1 or 2 scallions, white and light green parts only, sliced

Directions:

1.   Preparing the Ingredients

2.   Heat the olive oil in a large soup pot over medium-high heat.

3.   Add the onion and cauliflower, and sauté for about 5 minutes, until the vegetables are slightly softened. Add the potatoes, water, and dried herbs, and season to taste with salt and pepper. Bring the soup to a boil, reduce the

heat to low, and cover the pot. Simmer for 15 to 20 minutes, until the potatoes are soft.

4.   Finish and Serve

5.   Using a hand blender, purée the soup until smooth. (Alternatively, let it cool slightly, then transfer to a countertop blender.) Stir in the scallions and serve. Leftovers will keep in an airtight container for up to 1 week in the refrigerator or up to 1 month in the freezer.

Nutrition Info: Per Serving: (2 cups) Calories 80; Protein: 2g; Total fat: 1g; Saturated fat: 0g; Carbohydrates: 17g; Fiber: 3g

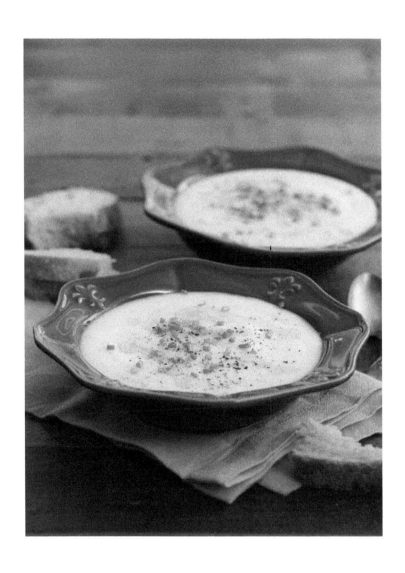

Rice Noodle Soup with Beans

Servings: 6

Cooking Time: 10 Minutes

Ingredients:

- 2 carrots, chopped
- 2 celery stalks, chopped
- 6 cups vegetable broth
- 8 oz brown rice noodles
- 1 (15-oz) can pinto beans
- 1 tsp dried herbs

Directions:

1. Place a pot over medium heat and add in the carrots, celery and vegetable broth. Bring to a boil. Add in noodles, beans, dried herbs, salt, and pepper. Reduce the heat and simmer for 5 minutes. Serve.

Hot Lentil Soup with Zucchini

Servings: 4

Cooking Time: 30 Minutes

Ingredients:

- 2 tbsp olive oil
- 1 onion, chopped
- 1 zucchini, chopped
- 1 garlic clove, minced
- 1 tbsp hot paprika
- 1 (14.5-oz) can crushed tomatoes
- 1 cup red lentils, rinsed
- 4 cups vegetable broth
- 3 cups chopped Swiss chard

Directions:

1.	Heat the oil in a pot over medium heat. Place in onion, zucchini, and garlic and sauté for 5 minutes until tender. Add in paprika, tomatoes, lentils, broth, salt, and pepper. Bring to a boil, then lower the heat and simmer for minutes, stirring often. Add in the Swiss chard and cook for another 3-5 minutes. Serve immediately.

Moroccan Vermicelli Vegetable Soup

Servings: 4 To 6

Cooking Time: 35 Minutes

Ingredients:

- 1 tablespoon extra-virgin olive oil
- 1 small onion, chopped
- 1 large carrot, chopped
- 1 celery rib, chopped
- 3 small zucchini, cut into 1/4-inch dice
- 1 (28-ounce) can diced tomatoes, drained
- 2 tablespoons tomato paste
- 1½cups cooked or 1 (15.5-ounce) can chickpeas, drained and rinsed
- 2 teaspoons smoked paprika
- 1 teaspoon ground cumin
- 1 teaspoon za'atar spice (optional)
- ¼ teaspoon ground cayenne
- 6 cups vegetable broth, homemade or store-bought, or water
- Salt
- 4 ounces vermicelli
- 2 tablespoons minced fresh cilantro, for garnish

Directions:

1.   Preparing the Ingredients

2.   In a large soup pot, heat the oil over medium heat. Add the onion, carrot, and celery. Cover and cook until softened for about 5 minutes. Stir in the zucchini, tomatoes, tomato paste, chickpeas, paprika, cumin, za'atar, and cayenne. Add the broth and salt to taste. Bring to a boil, then reduce heat to low and simmer, uncovered, until the vegetables are tender for about 30 minutes.

3.   Finish and Serve

4.   Shortly before serving, stir in the vermicelli and cook until the noodles are tender for about 5 minutes. Ladle the soup into bowls, garnish with cilantro, then serve.

Pumpkin-pear Soup

Servings: 4

Cooking Time: 15 Minutes

Ingredients:

- 1 teaspoon extra-virgin olive oil or coconut oil
- 1 onion, diced, or 2 teaspoons onion powder
- 1-inch piece fresh ginger, peeled and diced, or 1 teaspoon ground ginger
- 1 pear, cored and chopped
- Optional spices to take the taste up a notch:
- 1 teaspoon curry powder
- ½ teaspoon pumpkin pie spice
- ½ teaspoon smoked paprika
- Pinch red pepper flakes
- 4 cups water or Vegetable Broth
- 3 cups canned pumpkin purée
- 1 to 2 teaspoons salt (less if using salted broth)
- Pinch freshly ground black pepper
- ¼ to ½ cup canned coconut milk (optional)
- 2 to 4 tablespoons nutritional yeast (optional)

Directions:

1. Preparing the Ingredients

2.   Heat the olive oil in a large pot over medium heat. Add the onion, ginger, and pear, then sauté for about 5 minutes until softened. Sprinkle in any optional spices and stir to combine.

3.   Add the water, pumpkin, salt, and pepper, then stir until smooth and combine. Cook until just bubbling for about 10 minutes.

4.   Finish and serve

5.   Stir in the coconut milk (if using) and nutritional yeast (if using), and remove the soup from the heat. Leftovers will keep in an airtight container for up to 1 week in the refrigerator, or up to 1 month in the freezer.

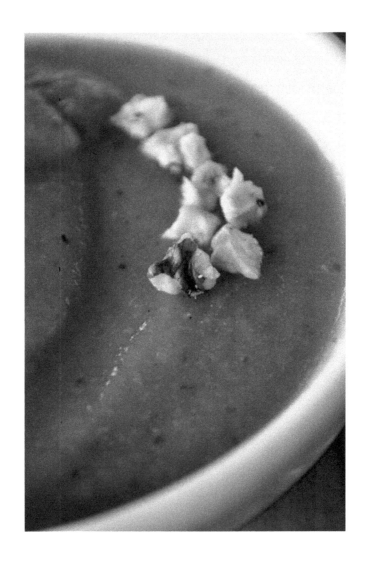

Old-fashioned Green Bean Salad

Servings: 4

Cooking Time: 10 Minutes

Ingredients:

- 1 ½ pounds green beans, trimmed
- 1/2 cup scallions, chopped
- 1 teaspoon garlic, minced
- 1 Persian cucumber, sliced
- 2 cups grape tomatoes, halved
- 1/4 cup olive oil
- 1 teaspoon deli mustard
- 2 tablespoons tamari sauce
- 2 tablespoons lemon juice
- 1 tablespoon apple cider vinegar
- 1/4 teaspoon cumin powder
- 1/2 teaspoon dried thyme
- Sea salt and ground black pepper, to taste

Directions:

1.   Boil the green beans in a large saucepan of salted water until they are just tender or about 2 minutes.

2.   Drain and let the beans cool completely; then, transfer them to a salad bowl. Toss the beans with the remaining ingredients.

3.   Bon appétit!

Nutrition Info: Per Serving: Calories: 240; Fat: 14.1g; Carbs: 29g; Protein: 4.4g

Pesto Pea Soup

Servings: 4

Cooking Time: 20 Minutes

Ingredients:

- 2 cups Water
- 8 oz. Tortellini
- ¼ cup Pesto
- 1 Onion, small & finely chopped
- 1 lb. Peas, frozen
- 1 Carrot, medium & finely chopped
- 1 ¾ cup Vegetable Broth, less sodium
- 1 Celery Rib, medium & finely chopped

Directions:

1. To start with, boil the water in a large pot over a medium-high heat.

2. Next, stir in the tortellini to the pot and cook it following the instructions given in the packet.

3. In the meantime, cook the onion, celery, and carrot in a deep saucepan along with the water and broth.

4. Cook the celery-onion mixture for 6 minutes or until softened.

5.   Now, spoon in the peas and allow it to simmer while keeping it uncovered.

6.   Cook the peas for few minutes or until they are bright green and soft.

7.   Then, spoon in the pesto to the peas mixture. Combine well.

8.   Pour the mixture into a high-speed blender and blend for 2 to 3 minutes or until you get a rich, smooth soup.

9.   Return the soup to the pan. Spoon in the cooked tortellini.

10.   Finally, pour into a serving bowl and top with more cooked peas if desired.

11.   Tip: If desired, you can season it with Maldon salt at the end.

Greek-style Roasted Pepper Salad

Servings: 2

Cooking Time: 10 Minutes

Ingredients:

- 2 red bell peppers
- 2 yellow bell peppers
- 2 garlic cloves, pressed
- 4 teaspoons extra-virgin olive oil
- 1 tablespoon capers, rinsed and drained
- 2 tablespoons red wine vinegar
- Seas salt and ground pepper, to taste
- 1 teaspoon fresh dill weed, chopped
- 1 teaspoon fresh oregano, chopped
- 1/4 cup Kalamata olives, pitted and sliced

Directions:

1.   Broil the peppers on a parchment-lined baking sheet for about minutes, rotating the pan halfway through the cooking time, until they are charred on all sides.

2.   Then, cover the peppers with a plastic wrap to steam. Discard the skin, seeds and cores.

3.   Slice the peppers into strips and place them in a salad bowl. Add in the remaining ingredients and toss to combine well.

4.   Place in your refrigerator until ready to serve. Bon appétit!

Nutrition Info: Per Serving: Calories: 185; Fat: 11.5g; Carbs: 20.6g; Protein: 3.7g

Cannellini Bean Soup with Kale

Servings: 5

Cooking Time: 25 Minutes

Ingredients:

* 1 tablespoon olive oil
* 1/2 teaspoon ginger, minced
* 1/2 teaspoon cumin seeds
* 1 red onion, chopped
* 1 carrot, trimmed and chopped
* 1 parsnip, trimmed and chopped
* 2 garlic cloves, minced
* 5 cups vegetable broth
* 12 ounces Cannellini beans, drained
* 2 cups kale, torn into pieces
* Sea salt and ground black pepper, to taste

Directions:

1.   In a heavy-bottomed pot, heat the olive over medium-high heat. Now, sauté the ginger and cumin for minute or so.

2.   Now, add in the onion, carrot and parsnip; continue sautéing an additional 3 minutes or until the vegetables are just tender.

3.   Add in the garlic and continue to sauté for 1 minute or until aromatic.

4.   Then, pour in the vegetable broth and bring to a boil. Immediately reduce the heat to a simmer and let it cook for 10 minutes.

5.   Fold in the Cannellini beans and kale; continue to simmer until the kale wilts and everything is thoroughly heated. Season with salt and pepper to taste.

6.   Ladle into individual bowls and serve hot. Bon appétit!

Nutrition Info: Per Serving: Calories: 188; Fat: 4.7g; Carbs: 24.5g; Protein: 11.1g

Thai Coconut Soup

Servings: 12

Cooking Time: 15 Minutes

Ingredients:

- 2 mangos, peeled, cut into bite-size pieces
- 1/2 cup green lentils, cooked
- 2 sweet potatoes, peeled, cubed
- 1/2 cup quinoa, cooked
- 1 green bell pepper, cored, cut into strips
- ½ teaspoon chopped basil
- ½ teaspoon chopped rosemary
- 2 tablespoons red curry paste
- 1/4 cup mixed nut
- 2 teaspoons orange zest
- 30 ounces coconut milk, unsweetened

Directions:

1. Take a large saucepan, place it over medium-high heat, add sweet potatoes, pour in the milk and bring the mixture to boil.

2. Then switch heat to medium-low level, add remaining ingredients, except for quinoa and lentils, stir and cook for 15 minutes until vegetables have softened.

3.   Then stir in quinoa and lentils, cook for minutes until hot, and then serve.

Nutrition Info: Calories: 232 Cal; Fat: 19.8 g: Carbs: 10.2 g; Protein: 7.8 g; Fiber: 0.8 g

Hearty Chili

Servings: 4

Cooking Time: 15 Minutes

Ingredients:

- 1 onion, diced
- 2 to 3 garlic cloves, minced
- 1 teaspoon extra-virgin olive oil, or 1 to 2 tablespoons water, vegetable broth, or red wine
- 1 (28-ounce) can tomatoes
- ¼ cup tomato paste, or crushed tomatoes
- 1 (14-ounce) can kidney beans, rinsed and drained, or 1½ cups cooked
- 2 to 3 teaspoons chili powder
- ¼ teaspoon sea salt
- ¼ cup fresh cilantro, or parsley leaves

Directions:

1. Preparing the Ingredients
2. In a large pot, sauté the onion and garlic in the oil for about 5 minutes. Once they're soft, add the tomatoes, tomato paste, beans, and chili powder. Season with the salt.

3.   Let it simmer for at least 10 minutes, or as long as you like. The flavors will get better the longer it simmers, and it's even better as leftovers.

4.   Finish and serve

5.   Garnish with cilantro and serve.

Nutrition Info: Per Serving: Calories: 160; Protein: 8g; Total fat: 3g; Saturated fat: 11g; Carbohydrates: 29g; Fiber: 7g

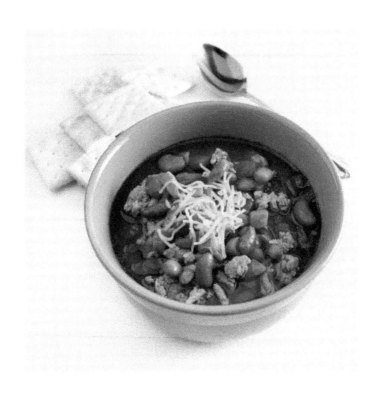

Ramen Noodle Soup

Servings: 2

Cooking Time: 20 Minutes

Ingredients:

- For The Mushrooms and Tofu:
- 2 cups sliced shiitake mushrooms
- 6 ounces tofu, extra-firm, drained, sliced
- 1 tablespoon olive oil
- 1 tablespoon soy sauce
- For the Noodle Soup:
- 2 packs of dried ramen noodles
- 1 medium carrot, peeled, grated
- 1 inch of ginger, grated
- 1 teaspoon minced garlic
- ¾ cup baby spinach leaves
- 1 tablespoon olive oil
- 6 cups vegetable broth
- For Garnish:
- Sesame seeds as needed
- Soy sauce as needed
- Sriracha sauce as needed

Directions:

1.	Prepare mushrooms and tofu and for this, place tofu pieces in a plastic bag, add soy sauce, seal the bag and turn it upside until tofu is coated.

2.	Take a skillet pan, place it over medium heat, add oil and when hot, add tofu slices and cook for 5 to 10 minutes until crispy and browned on all sides, flipping frequently and when done, set aside until required.

3.	Add mushrooms into the pan, cook for 8 minutes until golden, pour soy sauce from tofu pieces in it, and stir until coated.

4.	Meanwhile, prepare noodle soup and for this, take a soup pot, place it over medium-high heat, add oil and when hot, add garlic and ginger and cook for 1 minute until fragrant.

5.	Then pour in the broth, bring the mixture to boil, add noodles and cook until tender.

6.	Then stir spinach into the noodle soup, remove the pot from heat and distribute evenly between bowls.

7.	Add mushrooms and tofu along with garnishing and then serve.

Nutrition Info: Calories: 647 Cal; Fat: 12 g: Carbs: 106 g; Protein: 28 g; Fiber: 6 g

Classic Cream of Broccoli Soup

Servings: 4

Cooking Time: 35 Minutes

Ingredients:

- 2 tablespoons olive oil
- 1 pound broccoli florets
- 1 onion, chopped
- 1 celery rib, chopped
- 1 parsnip, chopped
- 1 teaspoon garlic, chopped
- 3 cups vegetable broth
- 1/2 teaspoon dried dill
- 1/2 teaspoon dried oregano
- Sea salt and ground black pepper, to taste
- 2 tablespoons flaxseed meal
- 1 cup full-fat coconut milk

Directions:

1.   In a heavy-bottomed pot, heat the olive oil over medium-high heat. Now, sauté the broccoli onion, celery and parsnip for about 5 minutes, stirring periodically.

2.   Add in the garlic and continue sautéing for 1 minute or until fragrant.

3.   Then, stir in the vegetable broth, dill, oregano, salt and black pepper; bring to a boil. Immediately reduce the heat to a simmer and let it cook for about 20 minutes.

4.   Puree the soup using an immersion blender until creamy and uniform.

5.   Return the pureed mixture to the pot. Fold in the flaxseed meal and coconut milk; continue to simmer until heated through or about minutes.

6.   Ladle into four serving bowls and enjoy!

Nutrition Info: Per Serving: Calories: 334; Fat: 24.5g; Carbs: 22.5g; Protein: 10.2g

Greek-style Pinto Bean and Tomato Soup

Servings: 4

Cooking Time: 30 Minutes

Ingredients:

- 2 tablespoons olive oil
- 1 carrot, chopped
- 1 parsnip, chopped
- 1 red onion, chopped
- 1 chili pepper, minced
- 2 garlic cloves, minced
- 3 cups vegetable broth
- 1 cup canned tomatoes, crushed
- 1/2 teaspoon cumin
- Sea salt and ground black pepper, to taste
- 1 teaspoon cayenne pepper
- 1 teaspoon Greek herb mix
- 20 ounces canned pinto beans
- 12 ounces canned corn, drained
- 2 tablespoons fresh cilantro, chopped
- 2 tablespoons fresh parsley, chopped
- 2 tablespoons Kalamata olives, pitted and sliced

Directions:

1.   In a heavy-bottomed pot, heat the olive over medium-high heat. Now, sauté the carrot, parsnip and onion for approximately 3 minutes or until the vegetables are just tender.

2.   Add in the chili pepper and garlic and continue to sauté for 1 minute or until aromatic.

3.   Then, add in the vegetable broth, canned tomatoes, cumin, salt, black pepper, cayenne pepper and Greek herb mix and bring to a boil. Immediately reduce the heat to a simmer and let it cook for 10 minutes.

4.   Fold in the beans and corn and continue simmering for about 10 minutes longer until everything is thoroughly heated. Taste and adjust the seasonings.

5.   Ladle into individual bowls and garnish with cilantro, parsley and olives. Bon appétit!

Nutrition Info: Per Serving: Calories: 363; Fat: 10.3g; Carbs: 55.2g; Protein: 17g

Avocado Mint Soup

Servings: 2

Cooking Time: 10 Minutes

Ingredients:

- 1 medium avocado, peeled, pitted, and cut into pieces
- 1 cup coconut milk
- 2 romaine lettuce leaves
- 20 fresh mint leaves
- 1 tbsp fresh lime juice
- 1/8 tsp salt

Directions:

1. Add all ingredients into the blender and blend until smooth. Soup should be thick not as a puree.
2. Pour into the serving bowls and place in the refrigerator for 10 minutes.
3. Stir well and serve chilled.

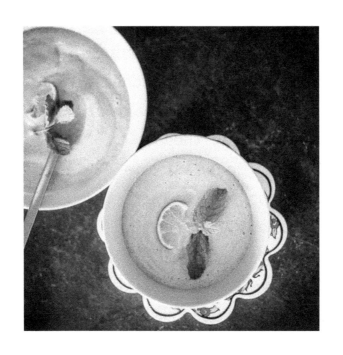

Mom's Cauliflower Coleslaw

Servings: 4

Cooking Time: 10 Minutes

Ingredients:

- 2 cups small cauliflower florets, frozen and thawed
- 2 cups red cabbage, shredded
- 1 cup carrots, trimmed and shredded
- 1 medium onion, chopped
- 1/2 cup vegan mayonnaise
- 4 tablespoons coconut yogurt, unsweetened
- 1 tablespoon yellow mustard
- 1 tablespoon fresh lemon juice
- 1/2 teaspoon cayenne pepper
- Sea salt and ground black pepper, to taste

Directions:

1. In a salad bowl, toss the vegetables until well combined.

2. In a small mixing bowl, thoroughly combine the remaining ingredients. Add the mayo dressing to the vegetables and toss to combine well.

3. Place the coleslaw in your refrigerator until ready to serve. Bon appétit!

Nutrition Info: Per Serving: Calories: 280; Fat: 24.6g; Carbs: 13.8g; Protein: 3.3g

Indian-style Naan Salad

Servings: 3

Cooking Time: 10 Minutes

Ingredients:

- 3 tablespoons sesame oil
- 1 teaspoon ginger, peeled and minced
- 1/2 teaspoon cumin seeds
- 1/2 teaspoon mustard seeds
- 1/2 teaspoon mixed peppercorns
- 1 tablespoon curry leaves
- 3 naan breads, broken into bite-sized pieces
- 1 shallot, chopped
- 2 tomatoes, chopped
- Himalayan salt, to taste
- 1 tablespoon soy sauce

Directions:

1. Heat 2 tablespoons of the sesame oil in a nonstick skillet over a moderately high heat.

2. Sauté the ginger, cumin seeds, mustard seeds, mixed peppercorns and curry leaves for 1 minute or so, until fragrant.

3.   Stir in the naan breads and continue to cook, stirring periodically, until golden-brown and well coated with the spices.

4.   Place the shallot and tomatoes in a salad bowl; toss them with the salt, soy sauce and the remaining 1 tablespoon of the sesame oil.

5.   Place the toasted naan on the top of your salad and serve at room temperature. Enjoy!

Nutrition Info: Per Serving: Calories: 328; Fat: 17.3g; Carbs: 36.6g; Protein: 6.9g

Easy Garbanzo Soup

Servings: 4

Cooking Time: 25 Minutes

Ingredients:

- 2 tbsp olive oil
- 1 onion, chopped
- 1 green bell pepper, diced
- 1 carrot, peeled and diced
- 4 garlic cloves, minced
- 1 (15-oz) can garbanzo beans
- 1 cup spinach, chopped
- 4 cups vegetable stock
- ¼ tsp ground cumin
- Sea salt to taste
- ¼ cup chopped cilantro

Directions:

1. Heat the oil in a pot over medium heat. Place in onion, garlic, bell pepper and carrot and sauté for 5 minutes until tender. Stir in garbanzo beans, spinach, vegetable stock, cumin, and salt. Cook for minutes. Mash the garbanzo using a potato masher, leaving some chunks. Top with cilantro and serve.

Celery Dill Soup

Servings: 4

Cooking Time: 25 Minutes

Ingredients:

- 2 tbsp coconut oil
- ½ lb celery root, trimmed
- 1 garlic clove
- 1 medium white onion
- ¼ cup fresh dill, roughly chopped
- 1 tsp cumin powder
- ¼ tsp nutmeg powder
- 1 small head cauliflower, cut into florets
- 3½ cups seasoned vegetable stock
- 5 oz. vegan butter
- Juice from 1 lemon
- ¼ cup coconut cream
- Salt and black pepper to taste

Directions:

1. Melt the coconut oil in a large pot and sauté the celery root, garlic, and onion until softened and fragrant, 5 minutes.

2.   Stir in the dill, cumin, and nutmeg, and stir-fry for 1 minute. Mix in the cauliflower and vegetable stock. Allow the soup to boil for 15 minutes and turn the heat off.

3.   Add the vegan butter and lemon juice, and puree the soup using an immersion blender.

4.   Stir in the coconut cream, salt, black pepper, and dish the soup.

5.   Serve warm.

Hot Bean & Corn Soup

Servings: 4

Cooking Time: 30 Minutes

Ingredients:

- 3 tbsp olive oil
- 1 onion, chopped
- 3 garlic cloves, chopped
- 1 cup sweet corn
- 1 (14.5-oz) can crushed tomatoes
- 1 (15.5-oz) can black beans
- 1 (4-oz) can chopped hot chilies
- 1 tsp ground cumin
- ½ tsp dried oregano
- 4 cups vegetable broth
- Salt and black pepper to taste
- ¼ cup chopped cilantro

Directions:

1.   Warm oil in a pot over medium heat. Place in the onion and garlic and sauté for 3 minutes. Add in sweet corn, tomatoes, beans, chilies, cumin, oregano, broth, salt, and pepper. Reduce the heat and simmer for

minutes. Divide between bowls and garnish with cilantro to serve.

Traditional Ukrainian Borscht

Servings: 4

Cooking Time: 40 Minutes

Ingredients:

- 2 tablespoons sesame oil
- 1 red onion, chopped
- 2 carrots, trimmed and sliced
- 2 large beets, peeled and sliced
- 2 large potatoes, peeled and diced
- 4 cups vegetable stock
- 2 garlic cloves, minced
- 1/2 teaspoon caraway seeds
- 1/2 teaspoon celery seeds
- 1/2 teaspoon fennel seeds
- 1 pound red cabbage, shredded
- 1/2 teaspoon mixed peppercorns, freshly cracked
- Kosher salt, to taste
- 2 bay leaves
- 2 tablespoons wine vinegar

Directions:

1.   In a Dutch oven, heat the sesame oil over a moderate flame. Once hot, sauté the onions until tender and translucent, about 6 minutes.

2.   Add in the carrots, beets and potatoes and continue to sauté an additional 10 minutes, adding the vegetable stock periodically.

3.   Next, stir in the garlic, caraway seeds, celery seeds, fennel seeds and continue sautéing for another seconds.

4.   Add in the cabbage, mixed peppercorns, salt and bay leaves. Add in the remaining stock and bring to boil.

5.   Immediately turn the heat to a simmer and continue to cook for 20 to 23 minutes longer until the vegetables have softened.

6.   Ladle into individual bowls and drizzle wine vinegar over it. Serve and enjoy!

Nutrition Info: Per Serving: Calories: 367; Fat: 9.3g; Carbs: 62.7g; Protein: 12.1g

Lightning Source UK Ltd.
Milton Keynes UK
UKHW020633140621
385477UK00005B/167